PLANT-BASED SJOGREN SYNDROME COOKBOOK FOR BEGINNERS

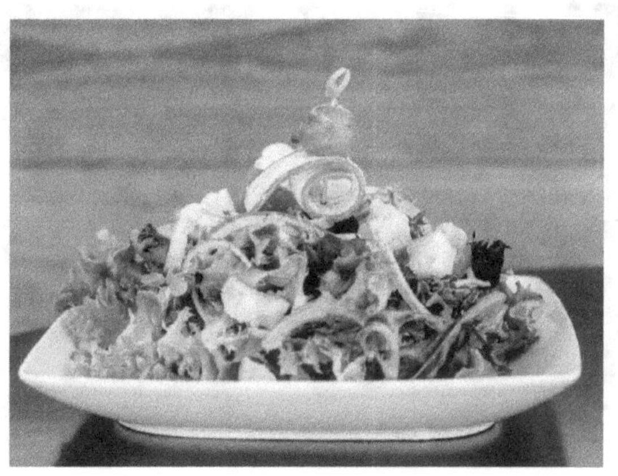

DR. JESSICA SMITH

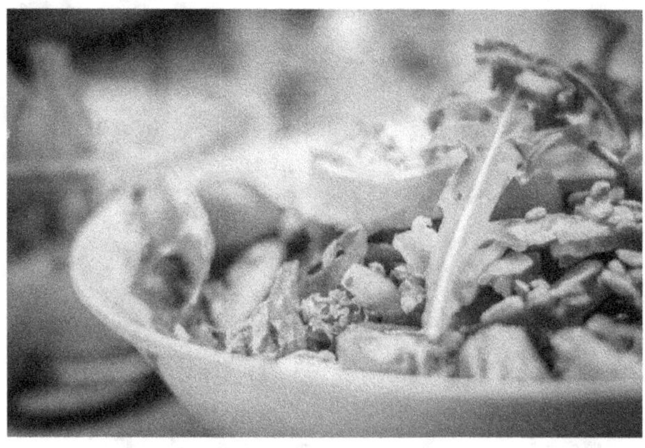

TABLE OF CONTENTS

CHAPTER ONE

How to Use this Cookbook

Familiarize Yourself with the Cookbook: Start by reading through the introduction and table of contents to get an overview of the cookbook's contents. Take note of any special features, such as meal plans, shopping lists, or nutritional information.

Gather Ingredients: Look through the recipes you'd like to try and make a list of the ingredients you'll need. Check your pantry and fridge to see what you already have and make a shopping list for anything you need to buy.

Plan Your Meals: Take some time to plan out your meals for the week using recipes from the cookbook. Consider factors like your schedule, dietary preferences, and any special occasions or events.

Start Simple: If you're new to plant-based cooking or cooking for Sjögren syndrome, start with simple recipes that use familiar ingredients and techniques. Look for recipes labeled as beginner-friendly or quick and easy.

Follow the Recipes Carefully: When cooking from the cookbook, follow the recipes closely, especially if you're unfamiliar with plant-based or Sjögren syndrome-specific cooking. Pay attention to measurements, cooking times, and any special instructions.

Experiment with Flavors: Don't be afraid to experiment with different herbs, spices, and seasonings to customize the recipes to your taste preferences. Add a pinch of garlic powder here or a dash of lemon juice there to enhance the flavors of your dishes.

Focus on Nutrient-Dense Foods: Look for recipes that emphasize nutrient-dense plant-based ingredients like fruits, vegetables, whole grains, legumes, nuts, and seeds. These foods are not only good for overall health but may also help manage symptoms of Sjögren syndrome.

Listen to Your Body: Pay attention to how your body responds to the plant-based meals you're eating. Notice if certain foods or ingredients seem to aggravate or alleviate your symptoms and adjust your meals accordingly.

Keep Track of Your Favorites: As you try different recipes from the cookbook, keep track of your favorites.

Consider creating a meal planning or recipe binder where you can store your favorite plant-based Sjögren syndrome recipes for easy reference.

Enjoy the Process: Cooking and eating plant-based meals can be a joyful and nourishing experience. Take pleasure in the process of preparing delicious, healthful meals for yourself and your loved ones, and savor the flavors and textures of the plant-based dishes you create.

Understanding Plant-Based Sjögren Syndrome for Beginners

Plant-based diets have gained popularity for their potential health benefits, including managing autoimmune conditions like Sjögren syndrome.

Sjögren syndrome is an autoimmune disorder that primarily affects the body's moisture-producing glands, leading to symptoms such as dry eyes, dry mouth, and fatigue.

While there is no cure for Sjögren syndrome, adopting a plant-based diet may help alleviate symptoms and improve overall well-being.

A plant-based diet focuses on whole, minimally processed foods derived from plants, such as fruits, vegetables, whole grains, legumes, nuts, and seeds.

These foods are rich in vitamins, minerals, antioxidants, and phytochemicals that support immune function, reduce inflammation, and promote overall health.

Additionally, plant-based diets are naturally low in saturated fat and cholesterol, which may help reduce the risk of heart disease, a common comorbidity in individuals with Sjögren syndrome.

For beginners looking to adopt a plant-based diet for Sjögren syndrome, it's essential to start by familiarizing themselves with plant-based foods and learning how to incorporate them into their meals.

This may involve experimenting with new recipes, exploring different cooking techniques, and gradually transitioning away from animal products.

Consulting with a healthcare provider or registered dietitian can also provide guidance and support in adopting a plant-based diet that meets individual nutritional needs and health goals.

Overall, understanding plant-based Sjögren syndrome for beginners involves recognizing the potential benefits of a plant-based diet in managing symptoms and improving overall health and well-being.

Principles of Plant-Based Sjögren Syndrome for Beginners

For beginners considering a plant-based approach to managing Sjögren syndrome, several key principles can guide them in adopting a healthful and sustainable lifestyle:

Emphasize Whole, Plant-Based Foods: Focus on incorporating a variety of whole, minimally processed plant foods into your diet, including fruits, vegetables, whole grains, legumes, nuts, and seeds.

These foods are rich in essential nutrients, antioxidants, and phytochemicals that can support overall health and help alleviate symptoms of Sjögren syndrome.

Prioritize Hydration: Since Sjögren syndrome often leads to dryness of the eyes and mouth, it's crucial to prioritize hydration.

Drink plenty of water throughout the day and include hydrating foods such as water-rich fruits and vegetables in your meals.

Opt for Anti-Inflammatory Foods: Certain plant foods, such as berries, leafy greens, nuts, and fatty fish (if included in your diet), have anti-inflammatory properties that may help reduce inflammation associated with Sjögren syndrome. Incorporating these foods into your meals can support overall health and well-being.

Limit or Avoid Trigger Foods: Some foods may exacerbate symptoms of Sjögren syndrome, such as those high in sugar, caffeine, alcohol, and processed ingredients. Pay attention to how your body responds to different foods and consider limiting or avoiding those that worsen your symptoms.

Practice Mindful Eating: Be mindful of your eating habits and listen to your body's hunger and fullness cues. Eat slowly, chew your food thoroughly, and savor the flavors and textures of plant-based meals.

By following these principles of plant-based Sjögren syndrome, beginners can lay a foundation for a healthful and nourishing diet that supports their overall well-being and helps manage their symptoms effectively.

Benefits of Plant-Based Sjogren Syndrome for Beginners

The benefits of adopting a plant-based diet for beginners managing Sjögren syndrome extend beyond mere nutrition, offering a holistic approach to symptom management and overall well-being. Here are several key advantages:

Reduced Inflammation: Plant-based diets are naturally rich in anti-inflammatory foods such as fruits, vegetables, nuts, seeds, and whole grains. By reducing inflammation in the body, individuals with Sjögren syndrome may experience relief from symptoms such as joint pain, fatigue, and dryness.

Improved Gut Health: Plant-based diets are typically high in fiber, which supports digestive health and promotes the growth of beneficial gut bacteria. A healthy gut microbiome is essential for immune function and may help alleviate gastrointestinal symptoms commonly associated with Sjögren syndrome, such as bloating and constipation.

Enhanced Hydration: Many plant-based foods have high water content, such as cucumbers, melons, and leafy greens. Consuming these hydrating foods can help alleviate symptoms of dryness associated with Sjögren syndrome by providing additional moisture to the body.

Heart Health Benefits: Plant-based diets are associated with a reduced risk of heart disease due to their low saturated fat and cholesterol content. By prioritizing plant-based foods, individuals with Sjögren syndrome can support cardiovascular health and reduce the risk of complications associated with heart disease.

Weight Management: Plant-based diets tend to be lower in calories and higher in fiber compared to omnivorous diets, making them an effective strategy for weight management. Maintaining a healthy weight is important for individuals with Sjögren syndrome as excess weight can exacerbate symptoms and increase the risk of complications.

Overall, adopting a plant-based diet offers numerous benefits for beginners managing Sjögren syndrome, including reduced inflammation, improved gut health, enhanced hydration, heart health benefits, and weight management support.

By incorporating more plant-based foods into their diet, individuals with Sjögren syndrome can optimize their health and well-being while effectively managing their symptoms.

Tips on Plant-Based Sjogren Syndrome for Beginners

For beginners embarking on a plant-based journey to manage Sjögren syndrome, here are some valuable tips to ease the transition and maximize the benefits:

Start Slowly: Transitioning to a plant-based diet can be overwhelming, so start by incorporating more plant-based meals gradually. Begin with one or two plant-based meals per day and gradually increase as you become more comfortable with the lifestyle.

Experiment with Flavors: Plant-based cooking offers a wide variety of flavors, textures, and cuisines to explore. Experiment with different herbs, spices, and seasonings to add excitement to your meals and keep your taste buds satisfied.

Focus on Whole Foods: Prioritize whole, minimally processed plant foods such as fruits, vegetables, whole grains, legumes, nuts, and seeds. These nutrient-dense foods provide essential vitamins, minerals, antioxidants, and fiber to support overall health and well-being.

Stay Hydrated: Sjögren syndrome often leads to dryness of the eyes and mouth, so it's essential to stay hydrated. Drink plenty of water throughout the day and include hydrating foods like watermelon, cucumber, and celery in your diet.

Plan Ahead: Planning your meals and snacks in advance can help you stay on track with your plant-based diet. Take some time each week to plan your meals, make a shopping list, and prepare ingredients ahead of time to streamline the cooking process.

Seek Support: Joining online communities or local support groups for plant-based eaters can provide valuable support, encouragement, and resources as you navigate your plant-based journey.

Surround yourself with like-minded individuals who can offer advice, share recipes, and provide motivation along the way.

Guidelines for beginners embracing a plant-based approach to managing Sjögren syndrome can provide structure and support as they navigate this new dietary journey:

Educate Yourself: Learn about the principles of plant-based nutrition and how it can benefit individuals with Sjögren syndrome. Understanding the rationale behind a plant-based diet can motivate and empower beginners to make informed choices.

Focus on Variety: Aim to include a wide variety of plant foods in your diet, including fruits, vegetables, whole grains, legumes, nuts, and seeds. This ensures you receive a diverse array of nutrients and phytochemicals that support overall health and symptom management.

Prioritize Hydration: Stay hydrated by consuming plenty of fluids throughout the day, including water, herbal teas, and hydrating fruits and vegetables. Adequate hydration is crucial for managing the dryness associated with Sjögren syndrome.

Monitor Nutrient Intake: Pay attention to your intake of key nutrients such as calcium, vitamin D, omega-3 fatty acids, and B vitamins, which may be of particular concern in a plant-based diet. Consider incorporating fortified foods or supplements as needed to meet your nutritional needs.

Listen to Your Body: Pay attention to how your body responds to different foods and adjust your diet accordingly. Notice any changes in symptoms or energy levels and make modifications as needed to support your overall well-being.

Consult a Healthcare Professional: Before making significant changes to your diet, consult with a healthcare professional or registered dietitian who can provide personalized guidance and support. They can help you develop a balanced plant-based eating plan that meets your individual needs and health goals.

By following these guidelines, beginners can embark on their plant-based journey with confidence, knowing they are taking proactive steps to manage their Sjögren syndrome while embracing a diet rich in nourishing, plant-based foods.

CHAPTER TWO

Plant-Based Sjogren Syndrome Recipes for
Beginners

1. Quinoa Salad

Ingredients:

- ➤ 1 cup quinoa
- ➤ 2 cups water or vegetable broth
- ➤ 1 cucumber, diced
- ➤ 1 bell pepper, diced
- ➤ 1 cup cherry tomatoes, halved
- ➤ 1/4 cup red onion, finely chopped
- ➤ 1/4 cup fresh parsley, chopped
- ➤ Juice of 1 lemon
- ➤ 2 tablespoons olive oil
- ➤ Salt and pepper to taste

Instructions:

- ➤ Rinse the quinoa under cold water.
- ➤ In a saucepan, bring the water or vegetable broth to
  a boil. Add quinoa, reduce heat, cover, and simmer

for 15-20 minutes or until liquid is absorbed and quinoa is fluffy.

➤ In a large bowl, combine cooked quinoa, cucumber, bell pepper, cherry tomatoes, red onion, and parsley.

➤ In a small bowl, whisk together lemon juice, olive oil, salt, and pepper. Pour over the salad and toss to combine.

➤ Serve chilled or at room temperature.

Health Benefits:

➤ Quinoa is rich in protein and fiber, which can help support digestive health and provide sustained energy.

➤ The vegetables provide essential vitamins and minerals, while olive oil offers healthy fats that are beneficial for heart health.

Preparation Time: 25 minutes

2. Lentil Soup

Ingredients:

➤ 1 cup dried lentils, rinsed

➤ 4 cups vegetable broth

- 1 onion, diced
- 2 carrots, diced
- 2 celery stalks, diced
- 2 garlic cloves, minced
- 1 teaspoon ground cumin
- 1 teaspoon paprika
- Salt and pepper to taste
- Fresh parsley for garnish (optional)

Instructions:

- In a large pot, combine lentils, vegetable broth, onion, carrots, celery, garlic, cumin, and paprika.
- Bring to a boil, then reduce heat to low and simmer for 20-25 minutes or until lentils and vegetables are tender.
- Season with salt and pepper to taste.
- Serve hot, garnished with fresh parsley if desired.

Health Benefits:

- Lentils are a good source of plant-based protein and are rich in fiber, which can help promote digestive health and regulate blood sugar levels.

- ➢ The vegetables in the soup provide essential nutrients and antioxidants.

Preparation Time: 30 minutes

3. Chickpea Stir-Fry

Ingredients:

- ➢ 1 can chickpeas, drained and rinsed
- ➢ 2 cups mixed vegetables (such as bell peppers, broccoli, carrots, and snap peas), chopped
- ➢ 2 cloves garlic, minced
- ➢ 1 tablespoon ginger, grated
- ➢ 2 tablespoons soy sauce or tamari
- ➢ 1 tablespoon maple syrup or agave nectar
- ➢ 1 tablespoon sesame oil
- ➢ Cooked brown rice or quinoa for serving

Instructions:

- ➢ Heat sesame oil in a large skillet over medium heat. Add garlic and ginger and sauté for 1 minute until fragrant.
- ➢ Add mixed vegetables to the skillet and stir-fry for 3-4 minutes until slightly tender.

➢ Add chickpeas, soy sauce, and maple syrup to the skillet. Stir well to combine and cook for another 2-3 minutes.

➢ Serve stir-fry over cooked brown rice or quinoa.

Health Benefits:

➢ Chickpeas are high in protein and fiber, which can help promote satiety and regulate blood sugar levels.

➢ The mixed vegetables provide a variety of vitamins, minerals, and antioxidants.

Preparation Time: 20 minutes

4. Spinach and Mushroom Stuffed Bell Peppers

Ingredients:

➢ 4 bell peppers, halved and seeds removed

➢ 2 cups spinach, chopped

➢ 1 cup mushrooms, chopped

➢ 1 onion, diced

➢ 2 cloves garlic, minced

➢ 1 cup cooked quinoa or brown rice

➢ 1 teaspoon dried oregano

- ➤ 1 teaspoon dried basil
- ➤ Salt and pepper to taste
- ➤ 1/2 cup marinara sauce
- ➤ 1/2 cup vegan cheese (optional)

Instructions:

- ➤ Preheat the oven to 375°F (190°C).
- ➤ In a large skillet, sauté onion and garlic over medium heat until softened.
- ➤ Add mushrooms to the skillet and cook until they release their moisture, about 5 minutes.
- ➤ Add spinach, cooked quinoa or brown rice, dried oregano, dried basil, salt, and pepper to the skillet. Cook until spinach is wilted.
- ➤ Spoon the mixture into halved bell peppers and place them in a baking dish.
- ➤ Top each stuffed pepper with marinara sauce and vegan cheese, if using.
- ➤ Cover the baking dish with foil and bake for 25-30 minutes, until peppers are tender.
- ➤ Remove foil and bake for an additional 5 minutes to melt the cheese, if using.

Health Benefits:

> - Bell peppers are rich in vitamin C, which can help support immune function and reduce inflammation.
> - Spinach and mushrooms are packed with vitamins, minerals, and antioxidants that promote overall health.

Preparation Time: 45 minutes

5. Sweet Potato and Black Bean Tacos

Ingredients:

> - 2 medium sweet potatoes, peeled and diced
> - 1 tablespoon olive oil
> - 1 teaspoon chili powder
> - 1/2 teaspoon ground cumin
> - Salt and pepper to taste
> - 1 can black beans, drained and rinsed
> - 1/2 cup corn kernels (fresh, canned, or frozen)
> - 1/4 cup red onion, diced
> - 1/4 cup fresh cilantro, chopped
> - 8 small corn or flour tortillas
> - Avocado slices, lime wedges, and hot sauce for serving

Instructions:

> ➤ Preheat the oven to 400°F (200°C).
> ➤ In a large bowl, toss diced sweet potatoes with olive oil, chili powder, cumin, salt, and pepper until evenly coated.
> ➤ Spread sweet potatoes in a single layer on a baking sheet and roast for 25-30 minutes, stirring halfway through, until tender and lightly browned.
> ➤ In a separate bowl, combine black beans, corn, red onion, and cilantro.
> ➤ Warm tortillas according to package instructions.
> ➤ Assemble tacos by filling each tortilla with roasted sweet potatoes and black bean mixture.
> ➤ Serve with avocado slices, lime wedges, and hot sauce.

Health Benefits:

> ➤ Sweet potatoes are a good source of vitamin A and fiber, which can help support eye health and promote digestive regularity.
> ➤ Black beans provide plant-based protein and fiber, while corn adds sweetness and additional fiber.

Preparation Time: 40 minutes

6. Vegan Buddha Bowl

Ingredients:

- 1 cup cooked quinoa
- 1 cup roasted sweet potatoes
- 1 cup steamed broccoli florets
- 1/2 cup shredded carrots
- 1/2 cup cooked chickpeas
- 1/4 cup sliced avocado
- 2 tablespoons tahini
- 1 tablespoon lemon juice
- 1 tablespoon water
- Salt and pepper to taste

Instructions:

- Arrange cooked quinoa, roasted sweet potatoes, steamed broccoli, shredded carrots, cooked chickpeas, and sliced avocado in a bowl.
- In a small bowl, whisk together tahini, lemon juice, water, salt, and pepper to make the dressing.
- Drizzle dressing over the Buddha bowl.
- Serve immediately.

Health Benefits:

> ➢ This Buddha bowl is packed with nutrient-dense ingredients, including quinoa, sweet potatoes, broccoli, carrots, chickpeas, and avocado, providing a wide range of vitamins, minerals, and antioxidants.
> ➢ Tahini adds healthy fats and a creamy texture to the dressing.

Preparation Time: 30 minutes

7. Vegan Tomato Basil Pasta

Ingredients:

> ➢ 8 oz (225g) whole wheat pasta
> ➢ 2 tablespoons olive oil
> ➢ 3 cloves garlic, minced
> ➢ 1 can (14 oz/400g) diced tomatoes
> ➢ 1/4 cup fresh basil, chopped
> ➢ Salt and pepper to taste
> ➢ Red pepper flakes (optional)

Instructions:

> ➢ Cook pasta according to package instructions. Drain and set aside.

➢ In a large skillet, heat olive oil over medium heat. Add minced garlic and sauté for 1-2 minutes until fragrant.

➢ Add diced tomatoes (with juices) to the skillet and simmer for 5-7 minutes until slightly thickened.

➢ Stir in chopped basil and cooked pasta. Season with salt, pepper, and red pepper flakes, if using.

➢ Toss to combine and cook for another 1-2 minutes.

➢ Serve hot, garnished with additional fresh basil if desired.

Health Benefits:

➢ Whole wheat pasta provides complex carbohydrates and fiber, which can help promote digestive health and provide sustained energy.

➢ Tomatoes are rich in vitamin C and lycopene, which have antioxidant properties and may help reduce inflammation.

Preparation Time: 20 minutes

8. Vegan Chickpea Curry

Ingredients:

- ➢ 1 tablespoon coconut oil
- ➢ 1 onion, diced
- ➢ 3 cloves garlic, minced
- ➢ 1 tablespoon grated ginger
- ➢ 1 tablespoon curry powder
- ➢ 1 teaspoon ground turmeric
- ➢ 1 can (14 oz/400g) diced tomatoes
- ➢ 1 can (14 oz/400g) coconut milk
- ➢ 2 cups cooked chickpeas
- ➢ 2 cups spinach
- ➢ Salt and pepper to taste
- ➢ Cooked brown rice or quinoa for serving

Instructions:

- ➢ Heat coconut oil in a large skillet over medium heat. Add diced onion and sauté until translucent.
- ➢ Add minced garlic, grated ginger, curry powder, and ground turmeric to the skillet. Cook for 1-2 minutes until fragrant.

- ➢ Stir in diced tomatoes (with juices) and coconut milk. Simmer for 10-15 minutes, stirring occasionally, until the sauce thickens.
- ➢ Add cooked chickpeas and spinach to the skillet. Cook for an additional 5 minutes until spinach is wilted.
- ➢ Season with salt and pepper to taste.
- ➢ Serve hot over cooked brown rice or quinoa.

Health Benefits:

- ➢ Chickpeas are a good source of plant-based protein and fiber, which can help promote satiety and regulate blood sugar levels.
- ➢ Spinach is rich in vitamins, minerals, and antioxidants that support overall health.

Preparation Time: 30 minutes

9. Vegan Banana Berry Smoothie Bowl

Ingredients:

- ➢ 2 ripe bananas, frozen
- ➢ 1 cup mixed berries (such as strawberries, blueberries, raspberries)

- ➤ 1/2 cup spinach or kale
- ➤ 1/2 cup unsweetened almond milk or coconut water
- ➤ Toppings: sliced bananas, mixed berries, granola, shredded coconut, chia seeds

Instructions:

- ➤ In a blender, combine frozen bananas, mixed berries, spinach or kale, and almond milk or coconut water.
- ➤ Blend until smooth and creamy, adding more liquid if needed to reach desired consistency.
- ➤ Pour smoothie into a bowl and top with sliced bananas, mixed berries, granola, shredded coconut, and chia seeds.
- ➤ Serve immediately.

Health Benefits:

- ➤ This smoothie bowl is packed with vitamins, minerals, and antioxidants from the bananas, mixed berries, and leafy greens.
- ➤ It's also rich in fiber and healthy fats from the toppings like granola, shredded coconut, and chia seeds.

Preparation Time: 10 minutes

10. Vegan Chocolate Avocado Mousse

Ingredients:

- ➤ 2 ripe avocados
- ➤ 1/4 cup cocoa powder
- ➤ 1/4 cup maple syrup or agave nectar
- ➤ 1 teaspoon vanilla extract
- ➤ Pinch of salt
- ➤ Fresh berries for serving (optional)

Instructions:

- ➤ Scoop the flesh of the avocados into a food processor.
- ➤ Add cocoa powder, maple syrup or agave nectar, vanilla extract, and a pinch of salt.
- ➤ Blend until smooth and creamy, scraping down the sides of the food processor as needed.
- ➤ Transfer the mousse to serving dishes and refrigerate for at least 30 minutes to chill.
- ➤ Serve topped with fresh berries if desired.

Health Benefits:

> ➢ Avocados are rich in healthy fats and fiber, which can help promote heart health and regulate blood sugar levels.
> ➢ Cocoa powder is a good source of antioxidants and may have anti-inflammatory properties.

Preparation Time: 10 minutes

11. Roasted Vegetable Quinoa Bowl

Ingredients:

> ➢ 1 cup quinoa
> ➢ 2 cups water or vegetable broth
> ➢ 1 small sweet potato, peeled and diced
> ➢ 1 zucchini, diced
> ➢ 1 red bell pepper, diced
> ➢ 1 yellow bell pepper, diced
> ➢ 1 tablespoon olive oil
> ➢ 1 teaspoon garlic powder
> ➢ 1 teaspoon smoked paprika
> ➢ Salt and pepper to taste
> ➢ 2 tablespoons tahini
> ➢ Juice of 1 lemon

➤ Fresh parsley for garnish (optional)

Instructions:

➤ Preheat the oven to 400°F (200°C).

➤ In a saucepan, bring water or vegetable broth to a boil. Add quinoa, reduce heat, cover, and simmer for 15-20 minutes or until liquid is absorbed and quinoa is fluffy.

➤ Place diced sweet potato, zucchini, and bell peppers on a baking sheet. Drizzle with olive oil and sprinkle with garlic powder, smoked paprika, salt, and pepper. Toss to coat.

➤ Roast vegetables in the preheated oven for 20-25 minutes, stirring halfway through, until tender and lightly browned.

➤ In a small bowl, whisk together tahini and lemon juice to make the dressing.

➤ To assemble the bowls, divide cooked quinoa among serving bowls. Top with roasted vegetables and drizzle with tahini dressing. Garnish with fresh parsley if desired.

➤ Serve warm.

Health Benefits:

> This bowl provides a variety of colorful vegetables rich in vitamins, minerals, and antioxidants, along with quinoa which is a good source of plant-based protein and fiber.
> Tahini adds healthy fats and a creamy texture to the dressing.

Preparation Time: 40 minutes

12. Coconut Curry Lentil Soup

Ingredients:

> 1 cup dried red lentils, rinsed
> 4 cups vegetable broth
> 1 can (14 oz/400ml) coconut milk
> 1 onion, diced
> 2 carrots, diced
> 2 cloves garlic, minced
> 1 tablespoon curry powder
> 1 teaspoon ground cumin
> 1 teaspoon ground turmeric
> Salt and pepper to taste
> Fresh cilantro for garnish (optional)

Instructions:

> In a large pot, combine red lentils, vegetable broth, coconut milk, onion, carrots, garlic, curry powder, cumin, turmeric, salt, and pepper.
> Bring to a boil, then reduce heat to low and simmer for 20-25 minutes, stirring occasionally, until lentils and vegetables are tender.
> Taste and adjust seasoning if needed.
> Serve hot, garnished with fresh cilantro if desired.

Health Benefits:

> Red lentils are rich in protein and fiber, which can help promote satiety and regulate blood sugar levels.
> Coconut milk adds creaminess and healthy fats to the soup, while the spices provide flavor and potential anti-inflammatory properties.

Preparation Time: 30 minutes

13. Mediterranean Chickpea Salad

Ingredients:

> 1 can chickpeas, drained and rinsed
> 1 cucumber, diced

- 1 cup cherry tomatoes, halved
- 1/4 cup red onion, thinly sliced
- 1/4 cup Kalamata olives, pitted and halved
- 2 tablespoons fresh parsley, chopped
- 2 tablespoons fresh mint, chopped
- Juice of 1 lemon
- 2 tablespoons extra virgin olive oil
- Salt and pepper to taste
- 2 oz (56g) vegan feta cheese, crumbled (optional)

Instructions:

- In a large bowl, combine chickpeas, cucumber, cherry tomatoes, red onion, Kalamata olives, parsley, and mint.
- In a small bowl, whisk together lemon juice, olive oil, salt, and pepper to make the dressing.
- Pour the dressing over the salad and toss to coat.
- If using, sprinkle vegan feta cheese over the salad before serving.
- Serve chilled or at room temperature.

Health Benefits:

> Chickpeas are rich in protein and fiber, while vegetables provide essential vitamins, minerals, and antioxidants.

> Olive oil is a source of healthy fats that can support heart health, and fresh herbs add flavor along with potential anti-inflammatory properties.

Preparation Time: 15 minutes

14. Stuffed Portobello Mushrooms

Ingredients:

> 4 large portobello mushrooms, stems removed

> 1 tablespoon olive oil

> 2 cloves garlic, minced

> 1/2 cup quinoa, cooked

> 1/2 cup cherry tomatoes, diced

> 1/4 cup sun-dried tomatoes, chopped

> 1/4 cup Kalamata olives, pitted and chopped

> 2 tablespoons fresh basil, chopped

> Salt and pepper to taste

> 1/4 cup vegan parmesan cheese (optional)

Instructions:

- ➢ Preheat the oven to 375°F (190°C).
- ➢ Place portobello mushrooms on a baking sheet lined with parchment paper.
- ➢ In a skillet, heat olive oil over medium heat. Add minced garlic and sauté for 1-2 minutes until fragrant.
- ➢ Add cooked quinoa, cherry tomatoes, sun-dried tomatoes, Kalamata olives, and fresh basil to the skillet. Cook for 2-3 minutes until heated through.
- ➢ Season the quinoa mixture with salt and pepper to taste.
- ➢ Spoon the quinoa mixture into the portobello mushrooms, dividing evenly.
- ➢ If using, sprinkle vegan parmesan cheese over the stuffed mushrooms.
- ➢ Bake in the preheated oven for 20-25 minutes until mushrooms are tender.
- ➢ Serve hot.

Health Benefits:

> Portobello mushrooms are a good source of B vitamins, selenium, and antioxidants.
> The quinoa filling provides protein and fiber, while tomatoes and olives add flavor along with vitamins, minerals, and healthy fats.

Preparation Time: 30 minutes

15. Vegan Lentil Shepherd's Pie

Ingredients:

> 2 cups cooked lentils
> 1 onion, diced
> 2 carrots, diced
> 2 celery stalks, diced
> 2 cloves garlic, minced
> 1 cup frozen peas
> 1 cup vegetable broth
> 2 tablespoons tomato paste
> 1 tablespoon soy sauce or tamari
> 1 teaspoon dried thyme
> 1 teaspoon dried rosemary
> Salt and pepper to taste

➢ 4 cups mashed potatoes (prepared in advance)

➢ Fresh parsley for garnish (optional)

Instructions:

➢ Preheat the oven to 375°F (190°C).

➢ In a large skillet, sauté onion, carrots, celery, and garlic over medium heat until softened.

➢ Add cooked lentils, frozen peas, vegetable broth, tomato paste, soy sauce, dried thyme, dried rosemary, salt, and pepper to the skillet. Stir well to combine.

➢ Simmer for 10-15 minutes until the mixture thickens slightly.

➢ Transfer the lentil mixture to a baking dish and spread mashed potatoes evenly on top.

➢ Bake in the preheated oven for 25-30 minutes until the top is golden brown.

➢ Serve hot, garnished with fresh parsley if desired.

Health Benefits:

➢ Lentils are a good source of plant-based protein and fiber, while vegetables provide essential vitamins, minerals, and antioxidants.

Preparation Time: 45 minutes

16. Tofu Stir-Fry

Ingredients:

- ➤ 14 oz (400g) firm tofu, pressed and cubed
- ➤ 2 tablespoons soy sauce or tamari
- ➤ 1 tablespoon sesame oil
- ➤ 1 tablespoon maple syrup or agave nectar
- ➤ 1 tablespoon cornstarch
- ➤ 2 tablespoons olive oil
- ➤ 1 bell pepper, sliced
- ➤ 1 cup broccoli florets
- ➤ 1 carrot, julienned
- ➤ 2 cloves garlic, minced
- ➤ 1 tablespoon grated ginger
- ➤ Cooked brown rice or quinoa for serving
- ➤ Sesame seeds for garnish (optional)
- ➤ Green onions, chopped, for garnish (optional)

Instructions:

- In a bowl, whisk together soy sauce, sesame oil, maple syrup or agave nectar, and cornstarch.
- Add cubed tofu to the bowl and toss to coat. Let marinate for 15-30 minutes.
- Heat olive oil in a large skillet or wok over medium heat. Add marinated tofu and cook until golden brown on all sides. Remove tofu from the skillet and set aside.
- In the same skillet, add bell pepper, broccoli, carrot, garlic, and ginger. Stir-fry for 5-7 minutes until vegetables are tender-crisp.
- Return tofu to the skillet and toss to combine with the vegetables.
- Serve stir-fry over cooked brown rice or quinoa.
- Garnish with sesame seeds and chopped green onions if desired.
- Serve hot.

Health Benefits:

- Tofu is a good source of plant-based protein and contains all nine essential amino acids.

> The colorful vegetables in this stir-fry provide vitamins, minerals, and antioxidants, while sesame oil adds flavor and healthy fats.

Preparation Time: 30 minutes

17. Vegan Broccoli Soup

Ingredients:

> 1 tablespoon olive oil
> 1 onion, diced
> 2 cloves garlic, minced
> 4 cups broccoli florets
> 3 cups vegetable broth
> 1 cup unsweetened almond milk or coconut milk
> Salt and pepper to taste
> Pinch of nutmeg (optional)
> Fresh chives for garnish (optional)

Instructions:

> In a large pot, heat olive oil over medium heat. Add diced onion and minced garlic. Sauté until onion is translucent.

- Add broccoli florets to the pot and cook for 2-3 minutes.
- Pour vegetable broth into the pot. Bring to a boil, then reduce heat and simmer for 10-15 minutes until broccoli is tender.
- Use an immersion blender to puree the soup until smooth. Alternatively, carefully transfer the soup to a blender and blend until smooth.
- Stir in almond milk or coconut milk. Season with salt, pepper, and nutmeg, if using.
- Serve hot, garnished with fresh chives if desired.

Health Benefits:

- Broccoli is rich in vitamins K and C, as well as fiber and antioxidants.
- This soup provides a comforting and nourishing meal, perfect for cooler days. Almond milk or coconut milk adds creaminess without dairy.

Preparation Time: 25 minutes

18. Vegan Stuffed Bell Peppers

Ingredients:

- ➤ 4 large bell peppers, tops removed and seeds removed
- ➤ 1 cup quinoa, cooked
- ➤ 1 can (14 oz/400g) black beans, drained and rinsed
- ➤ 1 cup corn kernels (fresh, canned, or frozen)
- ➤ 1/2 cup diced tomatoes
- ➤ 1/4 cup red onion, finely chopped
- ➤ 2 cloves garlic, minced
- ➤ 1 teaspoon chili powder
- ➤ 1 teaspoon ground cumin
- ➤ Salt and pepper to taste
- ➤ Fresh cilantro for garnish (optional)

Instructions:

- ➤ Preheat the oven to 375°F (190°C).
- ➤ In a large bowl, combine cooked quinoa, black beans, corn kernels, diced tomatoes, red onion, garlic, chili powder, cumin, salt, and pepper.
- ➤ Spoon the quinoa mixture into each bell pepper until filled.

➢ Place stuffed bell peppers in a baking dish. If necessary, slice a small portion from the bottom of each pepper to help them stand upright.

➢ Cover the baking dish with aluminum foil and bake in the preheated oven for 25-30 minutes, until peppers are tender.

➢ Remove foil and bake for an additional 5 minutes to lightly brown the tops.

➢ Serve hot, garnished with fresh cilantro if desired.

Health Benefits:

➢ Bell peppers are rich in vitamin C, fiber, and antioxidants, while quinoa and black beans provide plant-based protein and fiber.

➢ This dish is hearty and satisfying, perfect for a family dinner.

Preparation Time: 45 minutes

19. Vegan Banana Bread

Ingredients:

➢ 4 ripe bananas, mashed

➢ 1/4 cup coconut oil, melted

- 1/4 cup maple syrup or agave nectar
- 1 teaspoon vanilla extract
- 2 cups whole wheat flour
- 1 teaspoon baking powder
- 1/2 teaspoon baking soda
- 1/2 teaspoon ground cinnamon
- Pinch of salt
- 1/2 cup chopped walnuts or pecans (optional)

Instructions:

- Preheat the oven to 350°F (175°C). Grease a loaf pan and set aside.
- In a large bowl, combine mashed bananas, melted coconut oil, maple syrup or agave nectar, and vanilla extract.
- In a separate bowl, whisk together whole wheat flour, baking powder, baking soda, cinnamon, and salt.
- Gradually add the dry ingredients to the wet ingredients, stirring until just combined. Be careful not to overmix.
- Fold in chopped walnuts or pecans, if using.
- Pour the batter into the prepared loaf pan and smooth the top with a spatula.

- ➢ Bake in the preheated oven for 50-60 minutes, or until a toothpick inserted into the center comes out clean.
- ➢ Allow the banana bread to cool in the pan for 10 minutes before transferring to a wire rack to cool completely.
- ➢ Slice and serve.

Health Benefits:

- ➢ This banana bread is made with wholesome ingredients like ripe bananas, whole wheat flour, and coconut oil.
- ➢ It's naturally sweetened with maple syrup or agave nectar and contains no refined sugars or dairy.

Preparation Time: 1 hour

20. Vegan Chia Seed Pudding

Ingredients:

- ➢ 1/4 cup chia seeds
- ➢ 1 cup unsweetened almond milk or coconut milk
- ➢ 1 tablespoon maple syrup or agave nectar
- ➢ 1/2 teaspoon vanilla extract

- ➢ Fresh berries for serving
- ➢ Sliced almonds for serving

Instructions:

- ➢ In a bowl, combine chia seeds, almond milk or coconut milk, maple syrup or agave nectar, and vanilla extract. Stir well to combine.
- ➢ Cover the bowl and refrigerate for at least 4 hours or overnight, until the mixture thickens and becomes pudding-like in consistency.
- ➢ Stir the chia seed pudding before serving to redistribute the seeds.
- ➢ Divide the pudding into serving cups or bowls.
- ➢ Top with fresh berries and sliced almonds.
- ➢ Serve chilled.

Health Benefits:

- ➢ Chia seeds are rich in fiber, omega-3 fatty acids, and antioxidants.
- ➢ This pudding is a nutritious and satisfying snack or dessert option, providing a good balance of protein, healthy fats, and carbohydrates.

Preparation Time: 5 minutes (plus chilling time)

21. Vegan Lentil Sloppy Joes

Ingredients:

- 1 cup dried green lentils, rinsed
- 3 cups vegetable broth
- 1 onion, diced
- 2 cloves garlic, minced
- 1 bell pepper, diced
- 1 cup tomato sauce
- 2 tablespoons tomato paste
- 1 tablespoon maple syrup or agave nectar
- 1 tablespoon apple cider vinegar
- 1 tablespoon soy sauce or tamari
- 1 teaspoon chili powder
- 1/2 teaspoon smoked paprika
- Salt and pepper to taste
- Whole grain burger buns or bread rolls for serving

Instructions:

- In a large pot, combine lentils and vegetable broth. Bring to a boil, then reduce heat to low and simmer for 20-25 minutes, or until lentils are tender.

➢ In a skillet, heat olive oil over medium heat. Add diced onion, minced garlic, and diced bell pepper. Sauté until vegetables are softened.

➢ Add cooked lentils, tomato sauce, tomato paste, maple syrup or agave nectar, apple cider vinegar, soy sauce or tamari, chili powder, smoked paprika, salt, and pepper to the skillet. Stir well to combine.

➢ Simmer for 10-15 minutes, stirring occasionally, until the mixture thickens.

➢ Serve the lentil mixture on whole grain burger buns or bread rolls.

Health Benefits:

➢ Lentils are a good source of plant-based protein and fiber, which can help promote satiety and regulate blood sugar levels.

➢ This vegan twist on a classic comfort food is hearty and satisfying.

Preparation Time: 45 minutes

22. Vegan Spinach Artichoke Dip

Ingredients:

- 1 can (14 oz/400g) artichoke hearts, drained and chopped
- 2 cups fresh spinach, chopped
- 1 cup raw cashews, soaked in hot water for 1 hour and drained
- 1/4 cup nutritional yeast
- 2 cloves garlic, minced
- Juice of 1 lemon
- 1/4 teaspoon salt
- 1/4 teaspoon black pepper
- 1/4 teaspoon red pepper flakes (optional)
- Whole grain crackers, bread, or vegetable sticks for serving

Instructions:

- Preheat the oven to 375°F (190°C).
- In a food processor, combine chopped artichoke hearts, chopped spinach, soaked cashews, nutritional yeast, minced garlic, lemon juice, salt, pepper, and red pepper flakes if using.

- ➤ Pulse until the mixture is well combined but still slightly chunky.
- ➤ Transfer the mixture to a baking dish and spread it out evenly.
- ➤ Bake in the preheated oven for 20-25 minutes, until the dip is hot and bubbly.
- ➤ Serve hot with whole grain crackers, bread, or vegetable sticks for dipping.

Health Benefits:

- ➤ Spinach is rich in vitamins A and K, as well as iron and antioxidants.
- ➤ Cashews add creaminess and healthy fats to the dip, while nutritional yeast provides a cheesy flavor without dairy.

Preparation Time: 1 hour 30 minutes (including soaking time)

23. Vegan Cauliflower Buffalo Wings

Ingredients:

- ➤ 1 head cauliflower, cut into florets
- ➤ 1/2 cup all-purpose flour or chickpea flour

- ➢ 1/2 cup unsweetened almond milk or soy milk
- ➢ 1 teaspoon garlic powder
- ➢ 1 teaspoon onion powder
- ➢ 1/2 teaspoon smoked paprika
- ➢ Salt and pepper to taste
- ➢ 1/2 cup buffalo sauce
- ➢ Vegan ranch or blue cheese dressing for serving (optional)
- ➢ Celery sticks and carrot sticks for serving

Instructions:

- ➢ Preheat the oven to 450°F (230°C). Line a baking sheet with parchment paper.
- ➢ In a bowl, whisk together flour, almond milk or soy milk, garlic powder, onion powder, smoked paprika, salt, and pepper until smooth.
- ➢ Dip each cauliflower floret into the batter, coating evenly, then place it on the prepared baking sheet.
- ➢ Bake in the preheated oven for 20-25 minutes, until the cauliflower is golden brown and crispy.
- ➢ Remove the cauliflower from the oven and toss with buffalo sauce until evenly coated.

- ➤ Return the cauliflower to the baking sheet and bake for an additional 5 minutes.
- ➤ Serve hot with vegan ranch or blue cheese dressing, celery sticks, and carrot sticks for dipping.

Health Benefits:

- ➤ Cauliflower is low in calories and rich in vitamins and minerals, including vitamin C and potassium.
- ➤ This vegan version of buffalo wings is a healthier alternative to traditional chicken wings, with all the flavor and none of the guilt.

Preparation Time: 40 minutes

24. Vegan Coconut Curry Chickpea Stew

Ingredients:

- ➤ 1 tablespoon coconut oil
- ➤ 1 onion, diced
- ➤ 3 cloves garlic, minced
- ➤ 1 tablespoon grated ginger
- ➤ 1 tablespoon curry powder
- ➤ 1 teaspoon ground turmeric
- ➤ 1 can (14 oz/400g) diced tomatoes

- ➢ 1 can (14 oz/400ml) coconut milk
- ➢ 2 cups cooked chickpeas
- ➢ 2 cups chopped kale or spinach
- ➢ Salt and pepper to taste
- ➢ Cooked brown rice or quinoa for serving

Instructions:

- ➢ In a large pot, heat coconut oil over medium heat. Add diced onion and sauté until translucent.
- ➢ Add minced garlic, grated ginger, curry powder, and ground turmeric to the pot. Cook for 1-2 minutes until fragrant.
- ➢ Stir in diced tomatoes (with juices) and coconut milk. Simmer for 10-15 minutes, stirring occasionally.
- ➢ Add cooked chickpeas and chopped kale or spinach to the pot. Cook for an additional 5 minutes until greens are wilted.
- ➢ Season with salt and pepper to taste.
- ➢ Serve hot over cooked brown rice or quinoa.

Health Benefits:

> Chickpeas are a good source of plant-based protein and fiber, which can help promote satiety and regulate blood sugar levels.

> Kale and spinach are rich in vitamins, minerals, and antioxidants, while coconut milk adds creaminess and healthy fats.

Preparation Time: 30 minutes

25. Vegan Mediterranean Quinoa Salad

Ingredients:

> 1 cup quinoa

> 2 cups water or vegetable broth

> 1 cucumber, diced

> 1 cup cherry tomatoes, halved

> 1/4 cup red onion, thinly sliced

> 1/4 cup Kalamata olives, pitted and halved

> 1/4 cup fresh parsley, chopped

> 2 tablespoons fresh mint, chopped

> Juice of 1 lemon

> 2 tablespoons extra virgin olive oil

> Salt and pepper to taste

➤ 1/4 cup crumbled vegan feta cheese (optional)

Instructions:

➤ Rinse the quinoa under cold water.

➤ In a saucepan, bring the water or vegetable broth to a boil. Add quinoa, reduce heat, cover, and simmer for 15-20 minutes or until liquid is absorbed and quinoa is fluffy.

➤ In a large bowl, combine cooked quinoa, cucumber, cherry tomatoes, red onion, Kalamata olives, parsley, and mint.

➤ In a small bowl, whisk together lemon juice, olive oil, salt, and pepper to make the dressing.

➤ Pour the dressing over the salad and toss to coat.

➤ If using, sprinkle vegan feta cheese over the salad before serving.

➤ Serve chilled or at room temperature.

Health Benefits:

➤ Quinoa is a gluten-free whole grain rich in protein, fiber, and various vitamins and minerals.

➤ This salad is packed with fresh vegetables and herbs, providing essential nutrients and antioxidants. The addition of olives and olive oil adds healthy fats and flavor.

Preparation Time: 30 minutes

26. Vegan Ratatouille

Ingredients:

- ➢ 1 eggplant, diced
- ➢ 2 zucchini, diced
- ➢ 1 yellow squash, diced
- ➢ 1 onion, diced
- ➢ 2 cloves garlic, minced
- ➢ 1 bell pepper, diced
- ➢ 2 cups diced tomatoes
- ➢ 2 tablespoons tomato paste
- ➢ 1 teaspoon dried thyme
- ➢ 1 teaspoon dried oregano
- ➢ Salt and pepper to taste
- ➢ Fresh basil for garnish

Instructions:

- ➢ Preheat the oven to 375°F (190°C).

- In a large skillet, heat olive oil over medium heat. Add diced onion and minced garlic. Sauté until onion is translucent.
- Add diced eggplant, zucchini, yellow squash, and bell pepper to the skillet. Cook for 5-7 minutes, until vegetables start to soften.
- Stir in diced tomatoes, tomato paste, dried thyme, dried oregano, salt, and pepper. Cook for another 5 minutes.
- Transfer the mixture to a baking dish and spread it out evenly.
- Bake in the preheated oven for 25-30 minutes, until vegetables are tender.
- Serve hot, garnished with fresh basil.

Health Benefits:

- This classic French dish is packed with colorful vegetables rich in vitamins, minerals, and antioxidants.
- It's low in calories and high in fiber, making it a nutritious and satisfying meal.

Preparation Time: 45 minutes

27. Vegan Tofu Scramble

Ingredients:

- ➢ 14 oz (400g) firm tofu, drained and crumbled
- ➢ 1 tablespoon olive oil
- ➢ 1 onion, diced
- ➢ 1 bell pepper, diced
- ➢ 2 cups spinach or kale, chopped
- ➢ 2 cloves garlic, minced
- ➢ 1 teaspoon ground turmeric
- ➢ 1/2 teaspoon ground cumin
- ➢ Salt and pepper to taste
- ➢ Nutritional yeast for serving (optional)
- ➢ Whole grain toast or tortillas for serving

Instructions:

- ➢ Heat olive oil in a skillet over medium heat. Add diced onion and bell pepper. Sauté until softened.
- ➢ Add chopped spinach or kale and minced garlic to the skillet. Cook until greens are wilted.
- ➢ Push the vegetables to one side of the skillet and add crumbled tofu to the empty side.

- ➢ Sprinkle ground turmeric and ground cumin over the tofu. Stir well to combine with the vegetables.
- ➢ Cook for 5-7 minutes, stirring occasionally, until tofu is heated through and slightly browned.
- ➢ Season with salt and pepper to taste.
- ➢ Serve hot with nutritional yeast sprinkled on top, along with whole grain toast or tortillas.

Health Benefits:

- ➢ Tofu is a versatile plant-based protein that can be used as a substitute for scrambled eggs.
- ➢ This dish is high in protein and fiber, making it a satisfying breakfast or brunch option.

Preparation Time: 20 minutes

28. Vegan Pumpkin Soup

Ingredients:

- ➢ 1 tablespoon olive oil
- ➢ 1 onion, diced
- ➢ 2 cloves garlic, minced
- ➢ 4 cups diced pumpkin or butternut squash
- ➢ 4 cups vegetable broth

- 1 can (14 oz/400ml) coconut milk
- 1 teaspoon ground ginger
- 1/2 teaspoon ground cinnamon
- Salt and pepper to taste
- Pumpkin seeds for garnish (optional)
- Fresh parsley or cilantro for garnish (optional)

Instructions:

- In a large pot, heat olive oil over medium heat. Add diced onion and minced garlic. Sauté until onion is translucent.
- Add diced pumpkin or butternut squash to the pot. Cook for 5 minutes, stirring occasionally.
- Pour vegetable broth into the pot. Bring to a boil, then reduce heat and simmer for 15-20 minutes, until pumpkin is tender.
- Use an immersion blender to puree the soup until smooth. Alternatively, carefully transfer the soup to a blender and blend until smooth.
- Stir in coconut milk, ground ginger, ground cinnamon, salt, and pepper.
- Simmer for an additional 5 minutes, stirring occasionally.

> Serve hot, garnished with pumpkin seeds and fresh parsley or cilantro if desired.

Health Benefits:

> Pumpkin is rich in vitamins A and C, as well as fiber and antioxidants. This creamy soup is warming and comforting, perfect for chilly days.
> Coconut milk adds richness and healthy fats.

Preparation Time: 40 minutes

29. Vegan Spinach and Mushroom Stuffed Shells

Ingredients:

> 12 oz (340g) jumbo pasta shells
> 2 cups marinara sauce
> 1 tablespoon olive oil
> 1 onion, diced
> 2 cloves garlic, minced
> 8 oz (225g) mushrooms, sliced
> 4 cups fresh spinach
> 1 cup vegan ricotta cheese
> 1/4 cup nutritional yeast

- ➤ 1 teaspoon dried oregano
- ➤ 1 teaspoon dried basil
- ➤ Salt and pepper to taste
- ➤ Vegan mozzarella cheese for topping (optional)
- ➤ Fresh basil for garnish (optional)

Instructions:

- ➤ Preheat the oven to 375°F (190°C). Grease a baking dish and set aside.
- ➤ Cook jumbo pasta shells according to package instructions until al dente. Drain and set aside.
- ➤ In a skillet, heat olive oil over medium heat. Add diced onion and minced garlic. Sauté until onion is translucent.
- ➤ Add sliced mushrooms to the skillet. Cook until mushrooms are softened.
- ➤ Add fresh spinach to the skillet and cook until wilted.
- ➤ In a large bowl, combine vegan ricotta cheese, nutritional yeast, dried oregano, dried basil, salt, and pepper. Stir in the cooked mushroom and spinach mixture.
- ➤ Stuff each cooked pasta shell with the ricotta mixture and place them in the prepared baking dish.

- ➢ Pour marinara sauce over the stuffed shells, covering them evenly.
- ➢ If using, sprinkle vegan mozzarella cheese over the top.
- ➢ Cover the baking dish with aluminum foil and bake in the preheated oven for 20-25 minutes.
- ➢ Remove the foil and bake for an additional 5 minutes, until the cheese is melted and bubbly.
- ➢ Serve hot, garnished with fresh basil if desired.

Health Benefits:

- ➢ Spinach is rich in vitamins and minerals, while mushrooms provide additional nutrients and a meaty texture.
- ➢ This comforting dish is perfect for a family dinner or special occasion.

Preparation Time: 1 hour

30. Vegan Blueberry Oatmeal Muffins

Ingredients:

- ➢ 2 cups rolled oats
- ➢ 1 cup whole wheat flour

- 1/2 cup coconut sugar or brown sugar
- 2 teaspoons baking powder
- 1/2 teaspoon baking soda
- 1/2 teaspoon ground cinnamon
- 1/4 teaspoon salt
- 1 cup unsweetened applesauce
- 1/2 cup unsweetened almond milk or soy milk
- 1/4 cup coconut oil, melted
- 1 teaspoon vanilla extract
- 1 cup fresh or frozen blueberries

Instructions:

- Preheat the oven to 375°F (190°C). Line a muffin tin with paper liners or grease with oil.
- In a large bowl, combine rolled oats, whole wheat flour, coconut sugar or brown sugar, baking powder, baking soda, ground cinnamon, and salt.
- In a separate bowl, whisk together applesauce, almond milk or soy milk, melted coconut oil, and vanilla extract.
- Pour the wet ingredients into the dry ingredients and stir until just combined.
- Gently fold in blueberries.

- Divide the batter evenly among the muffin cups, filling each about 3/4 full.
- Bake in the preheated oven for 20-25 minutes, or until a toothpick inserted into the center comes out clean.
- Remove muffins from the oven and let cool in the tin for 5 minutes before transferring to a wire rack to cool completely.

Health Benefits:

- These muffins are made with wholesome ingredients like oats, whole wheat flour, applesauce, and blueberries.
- They're naturally sweetened and can be enjoyed as a nutritious breakfast or snack.

Preparation Time: 30 minutes

31. Vegan Lentil Meatballs

Ingredients:

- 1 cup dried green lentils, rinsed
- 3 cups vegetable broth
- 1 tablespoon olive oil

- 1 onion, finely chopped
- 2 cloves garlic, minced
- 1 teaspoon dried oregano
- 1 teaspoon dried basil
- 1/2 teaspoon smoked paprika
- 1/4 teaspoon red pepper flakes (optional)
- 1/4 cup tomato paste
- 1 cup breadcrumbs (gluten-free if needed)
- Salt and pepper to taste
- Marinara sauce for serving

Instructions:

- In a saucepan, combine lentils and vegetable broth. Bring to a boil, then reduce heat and simmer for 20-25 minutes, until lentils are tender and most of the liquid is absorbed.
- In a skillet, heat olive oil over medium heat. Add chopped onion and garlic. Sauté until onion is translucent.
- Add cooked lentils to the skillet along with dried oregano, dried basil, smoked paprika, and red pepper flakes if using. Cook for another 2-3 minutes.

- ➤ Transfer the mixture to a food processor. Add tomato paste and breadcrumbs. Pulse until well combined and the mixture comes together.
- ➤ Preheat the oven to 375°F (190°C). Line a baking sheet with parchment paper.
- ➤ Shape the lentil mixture into meatballs and place them on the prepared baking sheet.
- ➤ Bake in the preheated oven for 25-30 minutes, until meatballs are firm and lightly browned.
- ➤ Serve hot with marinara sauce over pasta or as a meatball sub.

Health Benefits:

- ➤ Lentils are an excellent source of plant-based protein and fiber, making these meatballs a nutritious alternative to traditional meatballs.
- ➤ They are also rich in essential vitamins and minerals, including folate, iron, and potassium.

Preparation Time: 1 hour

32. Vegan Chickpea Tacos

Ingredients:

- 1 can (14 oz/400g) chickpeas, drained and rinsed
- 1 tablespoon olive oil
- 1 onion, diced
- 2 cloves garlic, minced
- 1 teaspoon ground cumin
- 1 teaspoon chili powder
- 1/2 teaspoon smoked paprika
- Salt and pepper to taste
- 8 small corn tortillas
- Toppings: shredded lettuce, diced tomatoes, sliced avocado, chopped cilantro, lime wedges

Instructions:

- In a skillet, heat olive oil over medium heat. Add diced onion and minced garlic. Sauté until onion is translucent.
- Add drained chickpeas to the skillet along with ground cumin, chili powder, smoked paprika, salt, and pepper. Cook for 5-7 minutes, stirring

occasionally, until chickpeas are heated through and slightly crispy.

> Warm corn tortillas in a dry skillet or microwave.

> Assemble tacos by filling each tortilla with seasoned chickpeas and desired toppings.

> Serve hot with lime wedges for squeezing over the tacos.

Health Benefits:

> Chickpeas are a good source of plant-based protein, fiber, and essential nutrients.

> These tacos provide a satisfying and flavorful meal that is rich in vitamins, minerals, and antioxidants.

Preparation Time: 20 minutes

33. Vegan Sweet Potato and Black Bean Enchiladas

Ingredients:

> 2 large sweet potatoes, peeled and diced

> 1 tablespoon olive oil

> 1 onion, diced

> 2 cloves garlic, minced

- ➤ 1 can (15 oz/425g) black beans, drained and rinsed
- ➤ 1 teaspoon ground cumin
- ➤ 1 teaspoon chili powder
- ➤ Salt and pepper to taste
- ➤ 8 small corn tortillas
- ➤ 2 cups enchilada sauce
- ➤ 1 cup vegan shredded cheese
- ➤ Fresh cilantro for garnish

Instructions:

- ➤ Preheat the oven to 375°F (190°C). Grease a baking dish and set aside.
- ➤ Place diced sweet potatoes on a baking sheet. Drizzle with olive oil and toss to coat. Roast in the preheated oven for 20-25 minutes, until tender.
- ➤ In a skillet, heat olive oil over medium heat. Add diced onion and minced garlic. Sauté until onion is translucent.
- ➤ Add black beans to the skillet along with roasted sweet potatoes, ground cumin, chili powder, salt, and pepper. Cook for 5 minutes, stirring occasionally.
- ➤ Warm corn tortillas in a dry skillet or microwave.

- ➢ Spread a small amount of enchilada sauce on the bottom of the prepared baking dish.
- ➢ Place a spoonful of the sweet potato and black bean mixture in the center of each tortilla. Roll up and place seam-side down in the baking dish.
- ➢ Pour the remaining enchilada sauce over the rolled tortillas. Sprinkle vegan shredded cheese on top.
- ➢ Cover the baking dish with aluminum foil and bake in the preheated oven for 20-25 minutes, until the enchiladas are heated through and the cheese is melted.
- ➢ Serve hot, garnished with fresh cilantro.

Health Benefits:

- ➢ Sweet potatoes are rich in vitamins, minerals, and antioxidants, while black beans provide plant-based protein and fiber.
- ➢ These enchiladas are a satisfying and flavorful dish that is perfect for a family dinner or special occasion.

Preparation Time: 1 hour

34. Vegan Butternut Squash Risotto

Ingredients:

- 1 butternut squash, peeled, seeded, and diced
- 2 tablespoons olive oil, divided
- 1 onion, diced
- 2 cloves garlic, minced
- 1 1/2 cups Arborio rice
- 1/2 cup white wine (optional)
- 4 cups vegetable broth, heated
- Salt and pepper to taste
- 1/4 cup nutritional yeast (optional)
- Fresh parsley for garnish

Instructions:

- Preheat the oven to 400°F (200°C). Line a baking sheet with parchment paper.
- Place diced butternut squash on the prepared baking sheet. Drizzle with 1 tablespoon of olive oil and toss to coat. Roast in the preheated oven for 25-30 minutes, until tender and lightly browned.

- In a large skillet, heat the remaining 1 tablespoon of olive oil over medium heat. Add diced onion and minced garlic. Sauté until onion is translucent.
- Add Arborio rice to the skillet. Cook for 2-3 minutes, stirring constantly, until rice is lightly toasted.
- If using, pour white wine into the skillet. Cook until the wine is absorbed, stirring frequently.
- Gradually add heated vegetable broth to the skillet, 1/2 cup at a time, stirring constantly and allowing the liquid to be absorbed before adding more. Continue this process until the rice is creamy and tender, about 20-25 minutes.
- Stir in roasted butternut squash and nutritional yeast, if using. Season with salt and pepper to taste.
- Serve hot, garnished with fresh parsley.

Health Benefits:

- Butternut squash is rich in vitamins A and C, as well as fiber and antioxidants.
- Arborio rice provides a creamy texture without the need for dairy, making this risotto suitable for a plant-based diet.

Preparation Time: 1 hour

35. Vegan Chocolate Chia Seed Pudding

Ingredients:

- 1/4 cup chia seeds
- 1 cup unsweetened almond milk or coconut milk
- 2 tablespoons cocoa powder
- 2 tablespoons maple syrup or agave nectar
- 1/2 teaspoon vanilla extract
- Fresh berries for serving
- Shredded coconut for serving (optional)

Instructions:

- In a bowl, combine chia seeds, almond milk or coconut milk, cocoa powder, maple syrup or agave nectar, and vanilla extract. Stir well to combine.
- Cover the bowl and refrigerate for at least 4 hours or overnight, until the mixture thickens and becomes pudding-like in consistency.
- Stir the chia seed pudding before serving to redistribute the seeds.
- Divide the pudding into serving cups or bowls.

- Top with fresh berries and shredded coconut if desired.
- Serve chilled.

Health Benefits:

- Chia seeds are rich in fiber, omega-3 fatty acids, and antioxidants.
- This chocolate pudding is a nutritious and satisfying snack or dessert option, providing a good balance of protein, healthy fats, and carbohydrates.

Preparation Time: 5 minutes (plus chilling time)

36. Vegan Avocado Chocolate Mousse

Ingredients:

- 2 ripe avocados, peeled and pitted
- 1/4 cup cocoa powder
- 1/4 cup maple syrup or agave nectar
- 1/4 cup unsweetened almond milk or coconut milk
- 1 teaspoon vanilla extract
- Pinch of salt
- Fresh berries for serving
- Shredded coconut for serving (optional)

Instructions:

- Place avocados, cocoa powder, maple syrup or agave nectar, almond milk or coconut milk, vanilla extract, and salt in a blender or food processor.
- Blend until smooth and creamy, scraping down the sides as needed to ensure all ingredients are well combined.
- Divide the avocado chocolate mousse into serving cups or bowls.
- Cover and refrigerate for at least 30 minutes to chill and set.
- Serve chilled, topped with fresh berries and shredded coconut if desired.

Health Benefits:

- Avocados are rich in healthy fats, fiber, vitamins, and minerals.
- This chocolate mousse is a decadent and nutritious dessert option that is naturally sweetened and dairy-free.

Preparation Time: 10 minutes (plus chilling time)

37. Vegan Quinoa Salad with Roasted Vegetables

Ingredients:

- 1 cup quinoa
- 2 cups water or vegetable broth
- 1 sweet potato, peeled and diced
- 1 red bell pepper, diced
- 1 zucchini, diced
- 1 yellow squash, diced
- 1 red onion, diced
- 2 tablespoons olive oil
- 1 teaspoon smoked paprika
- 1/2 teaspoon garlic powder
- Salt and pepper to taste
- 1/4 cup chopped fresh parsley
- Balsamic vinaigrette for serving (optional)

Instructions:

- Rinse the quinoa under cold water.
- In a saucepan, bring the water or vegetable broth to a boil. Add quinoa, reduce heat, cover, and simmer for

15-20 minutes or until liquid is absorbed and quinoa is fluffy.

➢ Preheat the oven to 400°F (200°C). Line a baking sheet with parchment paper.

➢ In a large bowl, toss diced sweet potato, red bell pepper, zucchini, yellow squash, and red onion with olive oil, smoked paprika, garlic powder, salt, and pepper until well coated.

➢ Spread the vegetables in a single layer on the prepared baking sheet.

➢ Roast in the preheated oven for 20-25 minutes, stirring halfway through, until vegetables are tender and lightly browned.

➢ In a large bowl, combine cooked quinoa and roasted vegetables. Stir in chopped fresh parsley.

➢ Serve warm or at room temperature, drizzled with balsamic vinaigrette if desired.

Health Benefits:

➢ This quinoa salad is packed with nutrient-rich vegetables and whole grains, providing a balanced meal that is high in fiber, vitamins, and minerals.

➢ The roasted vegetables add depth of flavor and a satisfying texture.

Preparation Time: 45 minutes

38. Vegan Coconut Curry Tofu Stir-Fry

Ingredients:

➢ 14 oz (400g) firm tofu, pressed and cubed

➢ 2 tablespoons soy sauce or tamari

➢ 1 tablespoon sesame oil

➢ 1 tablespoon maple syrup or agave nectar

➢ 1 tablespoon cornstarch

➢ 2 tablespoons olive oil

➢ 1 bell pepper, sliced

➢ 1 cup broccoli florets

➢ 1 carrot, julienned

➢ 2 cloves garlic, minced

➢ 1 tablespoon grated ginger

➢ Cooked brown rice or quinoa for serving

➢ Sesame seeds for garnish (optional)

➢ Green onions, chopped, for garnish (optional)

Instructions:

> In a bowl, whisk together soy sauce, sesame oil, maple syrup or agave nectar, and cornstarch.

> Add cubed tofu to the bowl and toss to coat. Let marinate for 15-30 minutes.

> Heat olive oil in a large skillet or wok over medium heat. Add marinated tofu and cook until golden brown on all sides. Remove tofu from the skillet and set aside.

> In the same skillet, add bell pepper, broccoli, carrot, garlic, and ginger. Stir-fry for 5-7 minutes until vegetables are tender-crisp.

> Return tofu to the skillet and toss to combine with the vegetables.

> Serve stir-fry over cooked brown rice or quinoa.

> Garnish with sesame seeds and chopped green onions if desired.

> Serve hot.

Health Benefits:

> Tofu is a good source of plant-based protein and contains all nine essential amino acids.

> The colorful vegetables in this stir-fry provide vitamins, minerals, and antioxidants, while sesame oil adds flavor and healthy fats.

Preparation Time: 30 minutes

39. Vegan Lentil Shepherd's Pie

Ingredients:

- 2 cups cooked green lentils
- 1 onion, diced
- 2 cloves garlic, minced
- 2 carrots, diced
- 1 cup frozen peas
- 1 cup vegetable broth
- 2 tablespoons tomato paste
- 1 teaspoon dried thyme
- 1 teaspoon dried rosemary
- Salt and pepper to taste
- 4 cups mashed potatoes (prepared in advance)
- Fresh parsley for garnish (optional)

Instructions:

- Preheat the oven to 375°F (190°C).

> In a skillet, heat olive oil over medium heat. Add diced onion and minced garlic. Sauté until onion is translucent.

> Add diced carrots to the skillet and cook for 5 minutes, until slightly softened.

> Stir in cooked lentils, frozen peas, vegetable broth, tomato paste, dried thyme, dried rosemary, salt, and pepper. Cook for another 5 minutes, until heated through and the mixture thickens.

> Transfer the lentil mixture to a baking dish and spread it out evenly.

> Spread mashed potatoes over the lentil mixture in the baking dish.

> Bake in the preheated oven for 25-30 minutes, until the mashed potatoes are golden brown and the filling is bubbling.

> Serve hot, garnished with fresh parsley if desired.

Health Benefits:

> Lentils are a good source of plant-based protein and fiber, while vegetables provide vitamins, minerals, and antioxidants.

➢ This hearty shepherd's pie is a comforting and nutritious dish that is perfect for a cozy dinner.

Preparation Time: 1 hour

40. Vegan Banana Bread

Ingredients:

- ➢ 3 ripe bananas, mashed
- ➢ 1/4 cup coconut oil, melted
- ➢ 1/4 cup maple syrup or agave nectar
- ➢ 1 teaspoon vanilla extract
- ➢ 1 1/2 cups whole wheat flour
- ➢ 1 teaspoon baking soda
- ➢ 1/2 teaspoon ground cinnamon
- ➢ 1/4 teaspoon salt
- ➢ 1/2 cup chopped walnuts or pecans (optional)

Instructions:

- ➢ Preheat the oven to 350°F (175°C). Grease a 9x5-inch loaf pan and set aside.
- ➢ In a large bowl, combine mashed bananas, melted coconut oil, maple syrup or agave nectar, and vanilla extract.

- In a separate bowl, whisk together whole wheat flour, baking soda, ground cinnamon, and salt.
- Add the dry ingredients to the wet ingredients and stir until just combined. Fold in chopped walnuts or pecans if using.
- Pour the batter into the prepared loaf pan and smooth the top with a spatula.
- Bake in the preheated oven for 50-60 minutes, or until a toothpick inserted into the center comes out clean.
- Remove the banana bread from the oven and let cool in the pan for 10 minutes before transferring to a wire rack to cool completely.

Health Benefits:

- This banana bread is made with wholesome ingredients like whole wheat flour, bananas, and coconut oil.
- It's naturally sweetened and can be enjoyed as a delicious breakfast or snack.

Preparation Time: 1 hour

CONCLUSION

Embarking on a plant-based journey while managing Sjogren's syndrome can be a transformative and empowering experience.

By embracing the vibrant array of fruits, vegetables, grains, legumes, nuts, and seeds that nature provides, individuals with Sjogren's can nourish their bodies with nutrient-dense foods that support overall health and well-being.

This cookbook for beginners serves as a roadmap, guiding you through the process of creating delicious and satisfying plant-based meals that prioritize both flavor and functionality.

 From hearty soups to vibrant salads, from comforting stews to indulgent desserts, each recipe is thoughtfully crafted to provide nourishment and enjoyment.

But beyond the realm of taste, these recipes carry a deeper significance—they represent a commitment to self-care and compassion.

By choosing plant-based foods, we honor our bodies, our planet, and the animals with whom we share it.

We embrace a lifestyle that promotes longevity, vitality, and harmony with the world around us.

As you embark on your plant-based journey with Sjogren's syndrome, remember that it's not about perfection—it's about progress.

Every meal you prepare is a step toward better health, greater resilience, and a more sustainable future.

So, let this cookbook be your companion on this journey, inspiring you to explore new flavors, expand your culinary horizons, and thrive in every aspect of your life.

With each recipe you try, may you discover the joy of nourishing your body and soul with the goodness of plants.

And may your kitchen become a sanctuary—a place where healing and happiness intersect, and where every bite is a celebration of life itself.

Here's to your health, your happiness, and your journey toward wellness with Sjogren's syndrome. Bon appétit!